WILDERNESS SELF RELIANCE

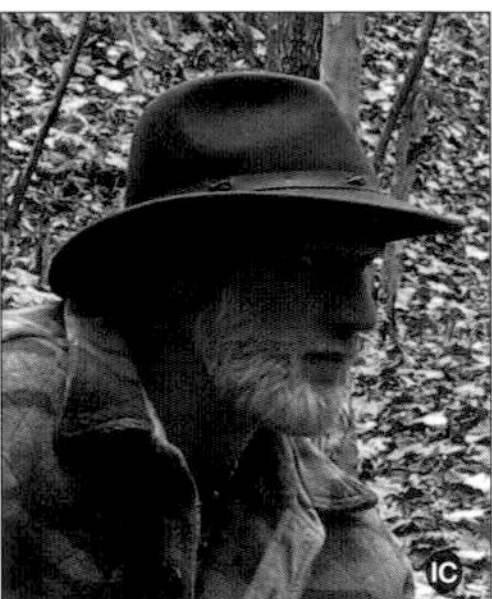

The Pathfinder School System®

Created as a teaching tool for my students in Wilderness Self Reliance, the Pathfinder School System represents the wisdom of the ancient scouts who ventured ahead of nomadic tribes to find fresh areas to support their community.

These "Pathfinders" had to accurately identify the perfect spot to sustain their tribes – they had to recognize the resources that would afford food, shelter, water, medicine and protection – the very same resources a person would need today.

In a survival situation, exertion and caloric output have to be constantly weighed against the caloric gain. Edible plants are often the most accessible and intelligent food choice, provided you are aware of a plant's nutritional value. Knowing which plants are edible and their relative caloric value is key to determining what to eat.

Not all plant food is of equal value, and very few plant foods (except nuts, seeds and grains) will offer the protein and fats you need for long-term strength. What they do offer, however, is a readily available source of carbohydrates, some fat and protein, and the all-important water that is essential for survival.

While this guide focuses on plants that are found in the eastern woodlands of the United States, these plants are likely to be found in other settings as well. You can survive with some of the basics outlined in this guide, but it is better if you have certain knowledge beforehand. Practice identifying species with trips to botanic gardens and garden shops.

What to Know

- **Pick 8 or 10 species** that are common to the wilderness areas that you visit, and learn to positively identify them.
- Select species that **do not have poisonous mimics.**
- Learn species that will be found in each of the seasons.
- Know which plant parts are edible, and how to prepare them.

Measurements refer to the height of plants unless otherwise indicated. The species are coded according to seasonal availability:

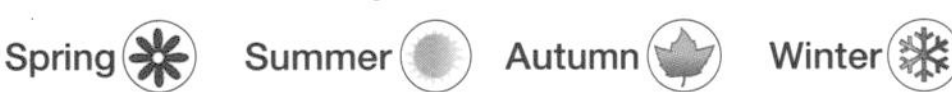
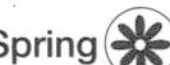
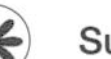
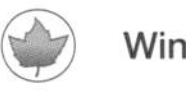

Spring Summer Autumn Winter

Dave Canterbury is a master woodsman with over 20 years of experience working in many dangerous environments. He has taught survival and survival methods to hundreds of students and professionals in the US and around the world. His common sense approach to survivability is recognized as one of the most effective systems of teaching known today. For information on Pathfinder programs and materials visit http://www.thepathfinderschoolllc.com.

Made in the USA

Waterford Press publishes reference guides that introduce readers to nature observation, outdoor recreation and survival skills. Product information is featured on the website: **www.waterfordpress.com**

To order or for information on custom published products please call 800-434-2555 or email orderdesk@waterfordpress.com. For permissions or to share comments email editor@waterfordpress.com.

ISBN 978-1-58355-707-5 $7.95 U.S.
50795
9 781583 557075
UPC 8 84682 00502 3
10 9 8 7 6 5 4 3 2 1 2206702

EDIBLE PLANTS OF THE EASTERN WOODLANDS – A Waterproof Folding Guide to Familiar Species

PATHFINDER OUTDOOR SURVIVAL GUIDE™

EDIBLE PLANTS OF THE EASTERN WOODLANDS

A Waterproof Folding Guide to Familiar Species

T0124013

THE PATHFINDER SCHOOL
www.thepathfinderschoolllc.com

EDIBLE WILD FOODS

An adult male typically needs about 18–20 calories per pound of body weight each day to remain healthy. Women need slightly fewer, and children/adolescents need slightly more. Survival situations, which are extremely stressful, can increase your caloric needs immensely since adrenalin is released as a result of stress and this causes the body to burn more calories.

All food contains 4 basic components: protein, fat, carbohydrates and water. Knowing which plant sources can satisfy your nutritional needs will help you in a survival situation.

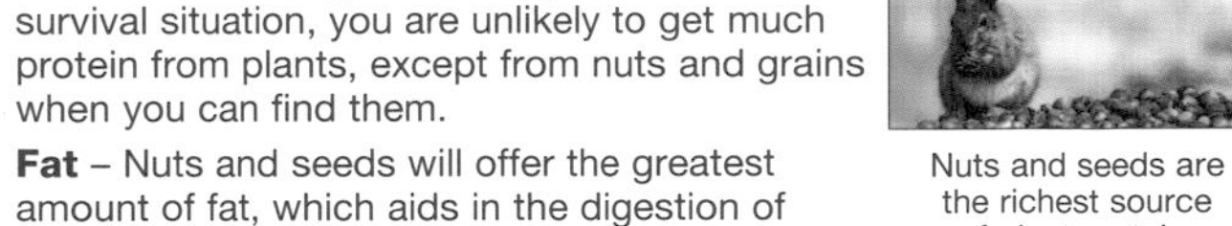

Nuts and seeds are the richest source of plant protein.

Protein – Plant proteins are generally 'incomplete', meaning you need to combine more than one to get a whole protein. In a survival situation, you are unlikely to get much protein from plants, except from nuts and grains when you can find them.

Fat – Nuts and seeds will offer the greatest amount of fat, which aids in the digestion of protein and provides energy.

Carbohydrates – Two main types of carbs are sugar and starch. Plant sources for carbs include fruits, berries, stocks/stems/roots (including some barks), nuts and seeds.

Water – Essential to all body functions, including digestion. Water is contained in plant foods in varying quantities. When drinking water is not easily obtained, consider the caloric cost of digestion before consuming foods with low nutritional value (mushrooms) or high-calorie foods that have little water content and take longer to digest (nuts, seeds).

Types of Edible Wild Plants

Roots & Tubers

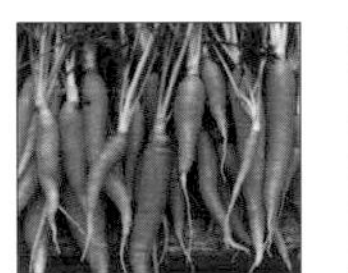

Taproot
Straight tapering root that grows downward.

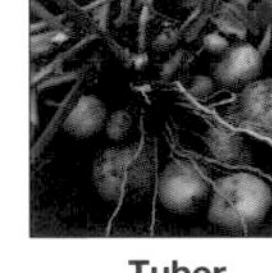

Tuber
An enlarged plant root.

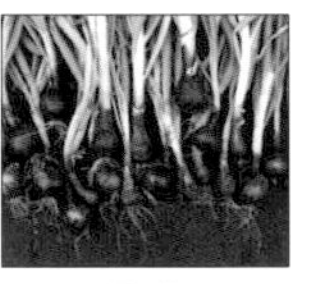

Bulb
An enlarged fleshy root of modified leaves.

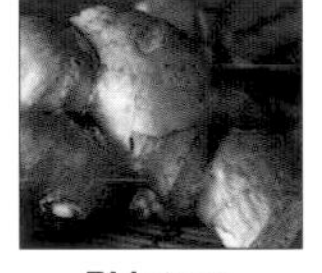
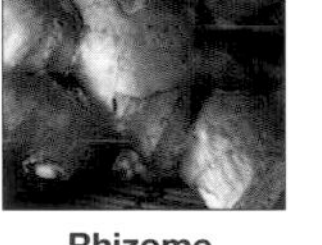

Rhizome
A plant stem that sends out roots from its nodes.

Fruits & Berries

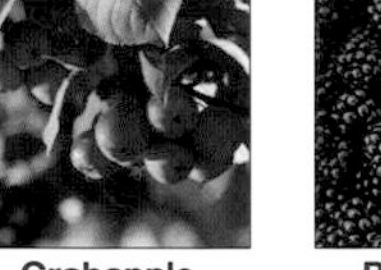

Crabapple

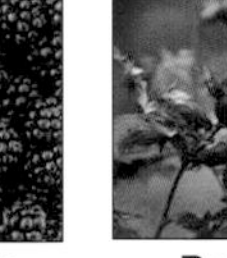

Blackberry

Rose Hip

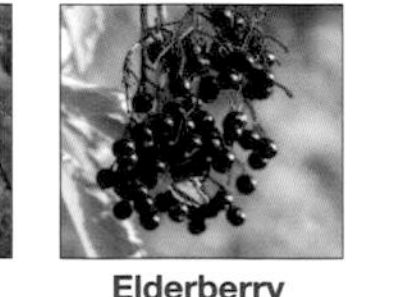

Elderberry

Nuts & Seeds

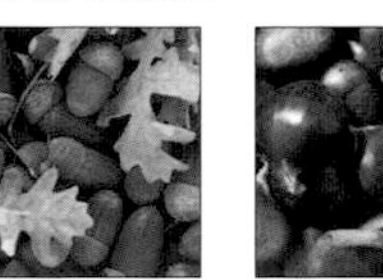

Acorns

Chestnuts, Walnuts

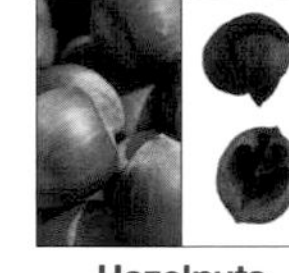

Hazelnuts, Hickory Nuts

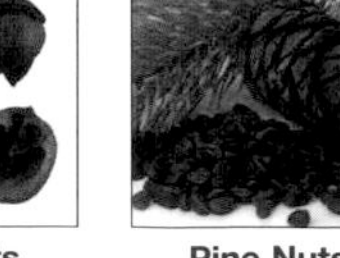

Pine Nuts
Small seed kernels are located under cone scales.

EDIBLE WILD FOODS

Stems & Leaves

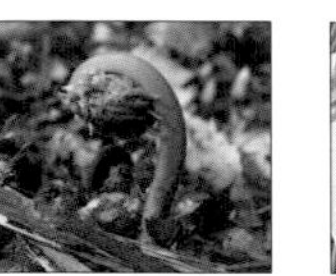

Shoots
Includes cattail, asparagus, some ferns (coiled fiddleheads in spring), bamboo.

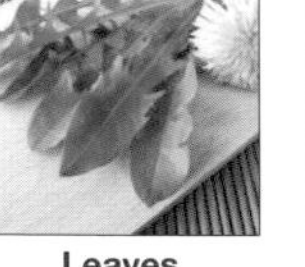
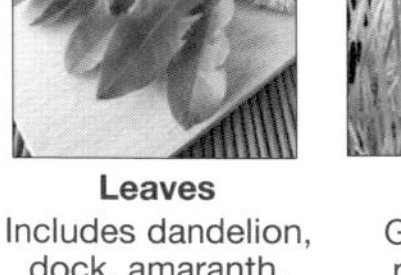

Leaves
Includes dandelion, dock, amaranth, plantain, onion, chicory, sorrel, some ferns.

Pith
Growth inside plant stem is edible in cattails, some palms and cacti, bamboo.

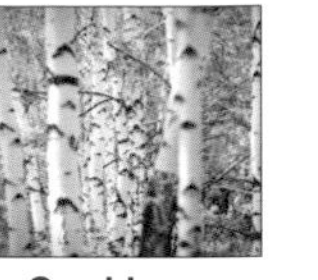

Cambium
Inner layer between the bark and the wood is edible in many conifers, birch, poplar, aspen.

SAFETY FIRST

The most important consideration when finding wild plant food is to avoid poisoning from toxic plants. Some – like poison ivy, poison oak and giant hogweed – are **toxic when handled** and can cause skin rashes and blistering. Others plants are **poisonous when eaten**. Eat only what you can absolutely positively identify and always conduct the universal edibility test before consuming wild plants.

- Never collect plants growing in contaminated water or from water that might contain parasites (like giardia). If you need to eat questionable plants, boil them in water for 15 minutes and discard the water.
- Some plants can develop fungal toxins – don't eat any fruit that shows signs of mildew or fungus.
- Signs of potentially poisonous plants include:
  - Milky sap
  - Seeds or beans inside pods
  - Bitter or soapy taste
  - Grains with pink to blackish spurs
  - Spines, thorns or fine hairs
  - Parsley or carrot-like foliage
  - Almond-scented
  - Leaves grow in 'threes'
- There are a few general rules to consider when determining if a berry is poisonous. The seeds of some – like chokecherry – contain cyanide and can kill you.
  - White, green and yellow berries are rarely edible.
  - Half of red berries are edible.
  - 90% of blue, black and purple berries are edible.
  - 99% of druplet fruits – raspberries, blackberries, etc. – are edible.
- Test all plant parts for edibility before you consume them. Some have both edible and inedible parts. Do not assume that a part that is edible when cooked is also edible when raw.
- Not all individuals react the same way to wild plants. Each person should individually test the plant part they are going to consume to ensure edibility and no reaction.
- As a rule, never eat wild mushrooms or any other fungi – they have little nutritional value and it is difficult to distinguish between edible and toxic varieties.

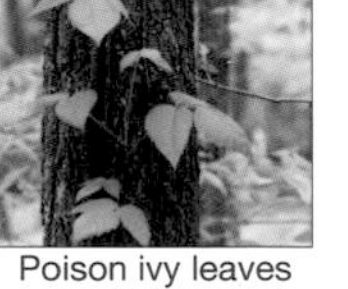

Poison ivy leaves grow in 'threes.'

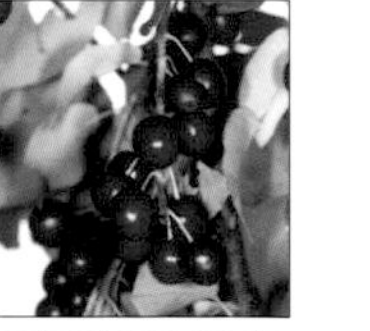

Chokecherry seeds contain cyanide.

SAFETY FIRST

Universal Edibility Test

1. **Separate the plant into its components** – leaves, stems, roots, buds/seeds/nuts/fruits/flowers. Test one plant part at a time.
2. **Smell the plant for strong or repellent odors.** Remember that the smell of almonds indicates the likelihood of a cyanide compound and should be avoided.
3. **Test for contact poisoning** by placing the plant piece that you are testing on the inside of your elbow or wrist. Usually you will see a reaction within 15 minutes.
4. **Select a small portion of the plant and prepare it the way you intend to eat it.** Before placing it in your mouth, do another safety check and touch a small portion to the outside of your lip to see if you react with burning or itching.
5. **If no reaction on the lip after 3 minutes,** hold a small amount in your mouth for 15 minutes (do not swallow it).
6. **If no itching, burning, swelling, numbing** or other irritation after 15 minutes, you can assume you have no reaction.
7. **If any reaction occurs,** induce vomiting immediately.
8. **If no ill effects after 8 hours, eat a small amount.** Wait another 8 hours and if no reaction, consider the food palatable to you.

NOTE: This edibility test is best done while you are learning about the plant species, rather than in a survival situation. Practice with known identified plants that you can obtain (don't use plants that have been treated with fertilizers or from roadsides or other polluted areas).

EASTERN WOODLANDS

The eastern woodlands is a region that encompasses three distinct forest types:

Temperate, Broadleaf & Mixed Forest
Forest biome is dominated by deciduous trees that lose their leaves in autumn. Dominant species include oaks, maples, hickories, beeches and elms.

Temperate Coniferous Forest
A mixed forest of conifers, evergreen broadleaf trees and deciduous broadleafs.

Flooded Grassland & Savanna
Dominant species include mangroves, cypresses, pines, palms, gum trees and figs.

Edible Plant Myths

- "If animals can eat it, so can I"....not true.
- "Boiling the plant in water will remove toxins" ... not always the case. If you have to eat it, follow the universal edibility test rules.
- "Plants with red parts are poisonous"...not always true, learn to identify species.

FORAGING TIPS

Fruits & Berries – An efficient way to harvest berries or fruit is to place a plastic sheet or tarp under a shrub or tree and shake it. Only ripe fruits will fall onto the sheet. If the fruits will not shake loose, make a 'rake' out of trimmed branches and drag along plant stems to harvest the berries.

Leaves, Shoots & Stems – As a rule, choose younger plants since these are generally more tender and tasty. Some plants are best picked by hand, while others, like chickweed, can be harvested by pulling the plant out of the ground and pulling the leaves off.

Roots & Tubers – Contain the most nutrients near the end of the growing season and are a good source of winter food. Cook like potatoes. Tough roots of species including cattails can be crushed to release starch and the dried liquid can be used as flour.

Nuts & Seeds – If water is in good supply, you can chop up nuts or seeds and immerse them. The shells will float and the seeds will sink. To winnow seeds from a seed head, simply rub the plant head back and forth between your hands over a shirt or tarp.

Removing Bitter Taste – Boiling in several changes of water will remove bitterness. If no fire or container to boil, put fruit or leaves in a cloth bag and submerge in clean stream or river for 1-3 days.

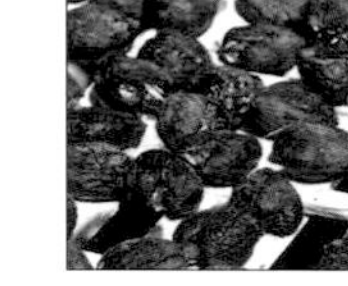

Drying – Fruits and nuts should be dried slowly away from direct heat or sunlight. Slice or crush roots, tubers and nuts and turn them over occasionally so they dry evenly and as quickly as possible.

PLANT PARTS

SIMPLE LEAF SHAPES

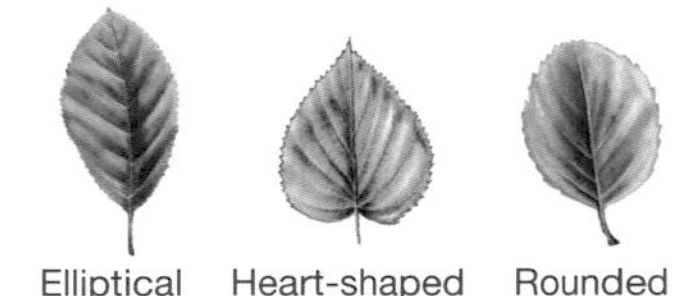
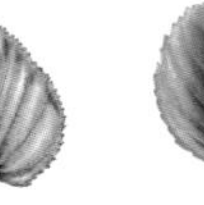
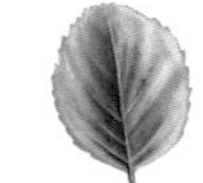
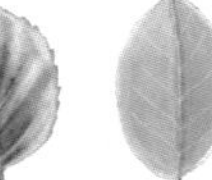

Elliptical, Heart-shaped, Rounded, Oval, Lobed, Lance-shaped

COMPOUND LEAVES

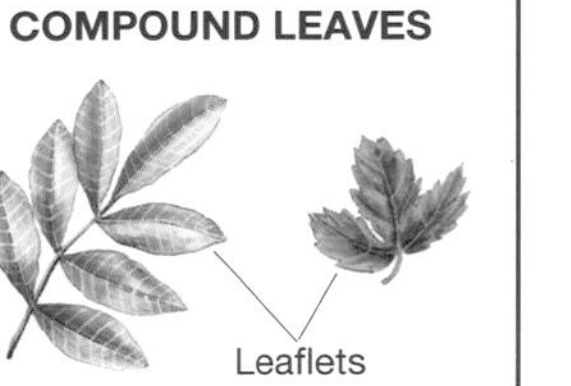

Leaflets

LEAF ARRANGEMENTS

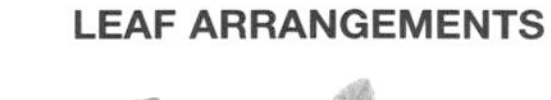
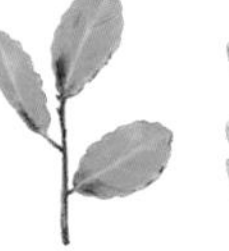
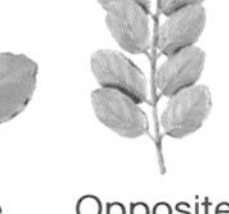
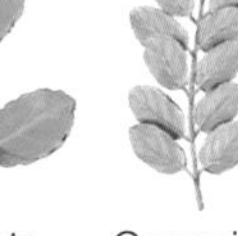
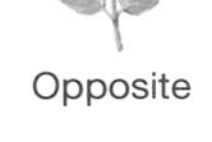

Alternate, Opposite, Whorled

FLOWER SHAPES

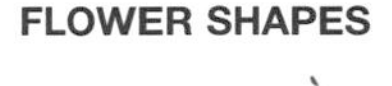
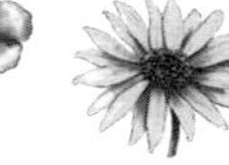
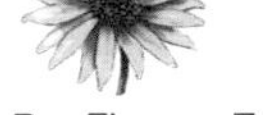
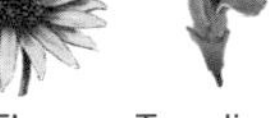
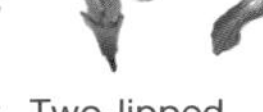
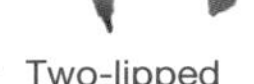
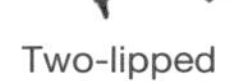

Bell, Cross, Trumpet, Ray Flower, Two-lipped, Iris, Pea-shaped

WILD EDIBLE PLANTS

Black Walnut
Juglans nigra
To 150 ft. (46 m)

Description: Alternate leaves have 9-21 leaflets. Flowers are succeeded by large, rounded fruits with a thick husk and a black, 4-celled nut inside.
Habitat: Mixed deciduous forests, bottomlands.
Harvest: Gather nuts in autumn.
Preparation: Allow nuts to dry to facilitate removing husk. Crush husks and remove nutmeats. Boil nuts for 30 minutes to leach out bitter flavor.
Comments: 3.5 oz. of nuts (about the weight of a 'D' battery) pack a whopping 628 calories of proteins, fat and carbohydrates.

Hickory
Carya spp.
To 80 ft. (24 m)

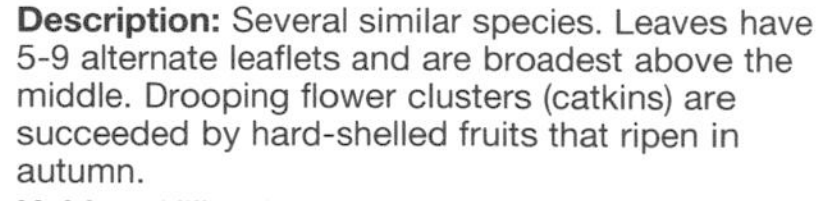

Description: Several similar species. Leaves have 5-9 alternate leaflets and are broadest above the middle. Drooping flower clusters (catkins) are succeeded by hard-shelled fruits that ripen in autumn.
Habitat: Hills, slopes, river valleys.
Harvest: Nutmeats from fruits. Put crushed nuts in boiling water and the nutmeats will float to the top and can be skimmed off.
Preparation: Eat raw or cooked.
Comments: The oil released by the nuts when they boil is also nutritious and should be skimmed off.

Oak
Quercus spp.
To 80 ft. (24 m)

Description: Several similar species. Leaf shapes are highly variable. All oaks produce distinctive, leathery, cup-shaped acorns that contain a single seed.
Habitat: Mixed deciduous forests, foothills, canyons.
Harvest: Nutmeats from fruits.
Preparation: Remove nutmeats. Bitterness of nutmeats can be tempered by soaking them for days in cool water (a stream is ideal) or boiling them in several changes of water.
Comments: Acorns vary in size from .5-2.5 in. and were one of the most important food sources relied upon by Native Americans.

Autumn Olive
Elaeagnus umbellata
To 15 ft. (4.5 m)

Description: Shrub or small tree has thorny branches. White to yellowish, tubular flowers are succeeded by juicy fruits.
Habitat: Riverbanks, meadows.
Harvest: Fruits.
Preparation: Eat raw or cooked.
Comments: Berries are an excellent source of the antioxidant lycopene.

Raspberry
Rubus spp.
To 6 ft. (1.8 m)

Description: Leaves have 3-7 leaflets. White to pinkish flowers are succeeded by the familiar bright red, druplet fruits.
Habitat: Woodland margins, roadsides, clearings.
Harvest: Fruits, shoots.
Preparation: Eat raw or cooked.
Comments: An excellent source of vitamins. Similar blackberries and salmonberries are also found in eastern woodlands.

WILD EDIBLE PLANTS

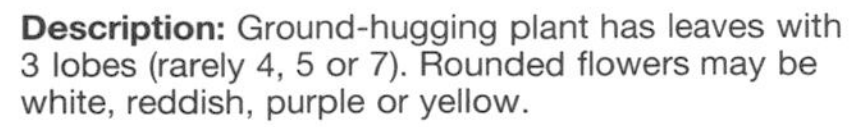
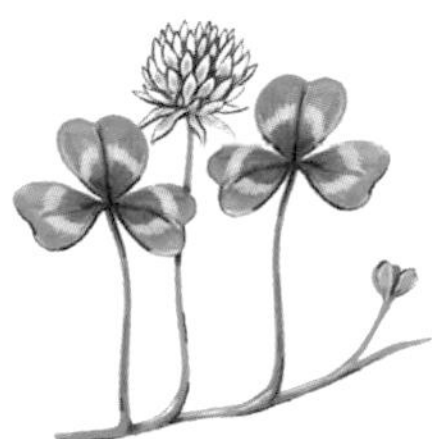

Clover
Trifolium spp.
Stems to 10 in. (25 cm)

Description: Ground-hugging plant has leaves with 3 lobes (rarely 4, 5 or 7). Rounded flowers may be white, reddish, purple or yellow.
Habitat: Open woodlands, meadows, fields.
Harvest: All parts of the plant are edible.
Preparation: Young leaves, flowers and roots can be eaten raw or boiled. Dried flower heads can be ground into flour.
Comments: About 20 of the 75 North American species grow in the eastern woodlands.

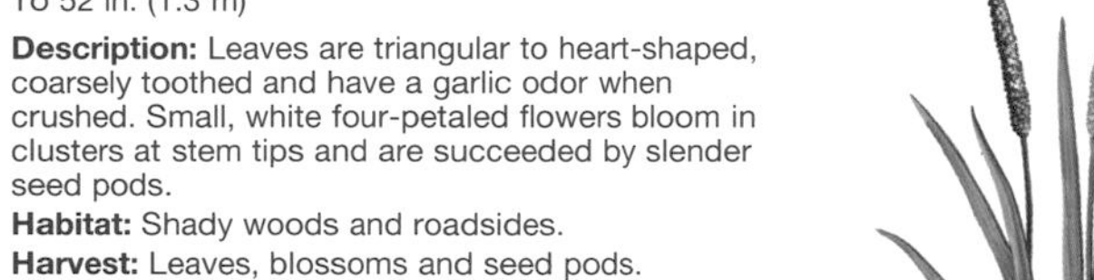

Garlic Mustard
Alliaria officinalis
To 52 in. (1.3 m)

Description: Leaves are triangular to heart-shaped, coarsely toothed and have a garlic odor when crushed. Small, white four-petaled flowers bloom in clusters at stem tips and are succeeded by slender seed pods.
Habitat: Shady woods and roadsides.
Harvest: Leaves, blossoms and seed pods.
Preparation: Eat raw or boiled.
Comments: Taproot smells like horseradish.

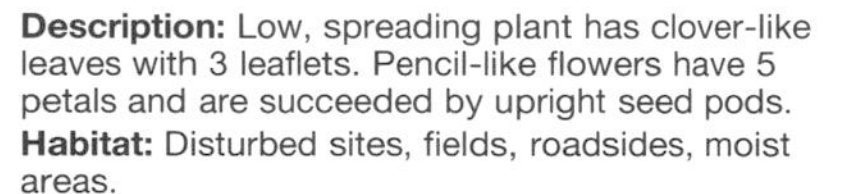

Yellow Wood Sorrel
Oxalis stricta
To 15 in. (38 cm)

Description: Low, spreading plant has clover-like leaves with 3 leaflets. Pencil-like flowers have 5 petals and are succeeded by upright seed pods.
Habitat: Disturbed sites, fields, roadsides, moist areas.
Harvest: Leaves, flowers, immature seed pods.
Preparation: Eat raw or boiled. Tea tastes like lemonade.
Comments: When ripe, the seed pods burst open at the slightest touch.

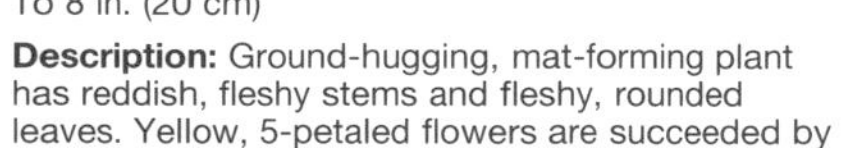

Purslane
Portulaca oleracea
To 8 in. (20 cm)

Description: Ground-hugging, mat-forming plant has reddish, fleshy stems and fleshy, rounded leaves. Yellow, 5-petaled flowers are succeeded by seed capsules.
Habitat: Fields, disturbed areas.
Harvest: Shoots, stems, leaves, seeds.
Preparation: Eat raw or boiled. Seeds can be dried and ground into flour.
Comments: Invasive weed has a high iron content. Flowers open in sunlight only.

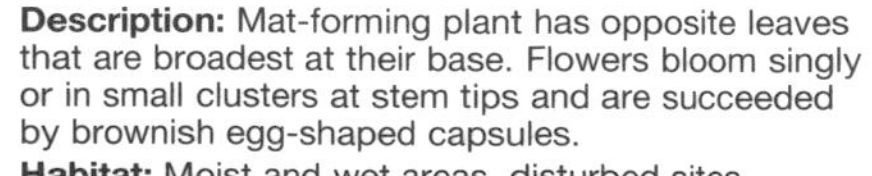

Common Chickweed
Stellaria media
To 12 in. (30 cm)

Description: Mat-forming plant has opposite leaves that are broadest at their base. Flowers bloom singly or in small clusters at stem tips and are succeeded by brownish egg-shaped capsules.
Habitat: Moist and wet areas, disturbed sites, woodlands.
Harvest: Leaves and stems.
Preparation: Eat raw or boiled.
Comments: A simple way to harvest the leaves and stems is to uproot the plant and cut off the leaves.

WILD EDIBLE PLANTS

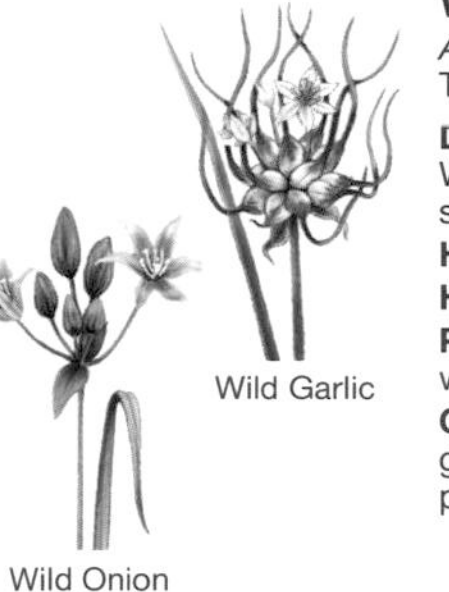

Wild Garlic

Wild Onion

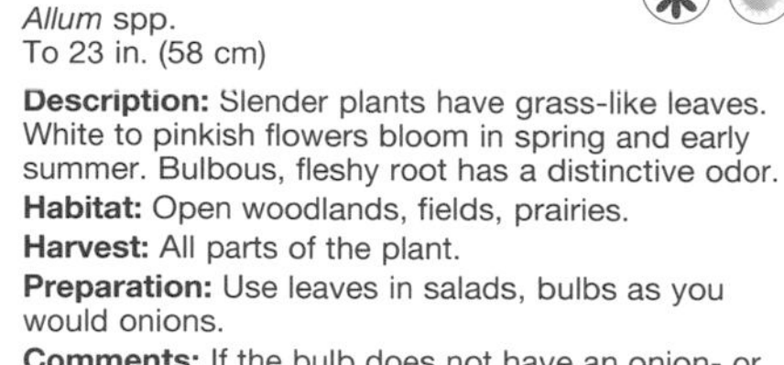

Wild Garlic & Wild Onion
Allum spp.
To 23 in. (58 cm)

Description: Slender plants have grass-like leaves. White to pinkish flowers bloom in spring and early summer. Bulbous, fleshy root has a distinctive odor.
Habitat: Open woodlands, fields, prairies.
Harvest: All parts of the plant.
Preparation: Use leaves in salads, bulbs as you would onions.
Comments: If the bulb does not have an onion- or garlic-like odor, do not eat it. Many similar-looking plants are poisonous.

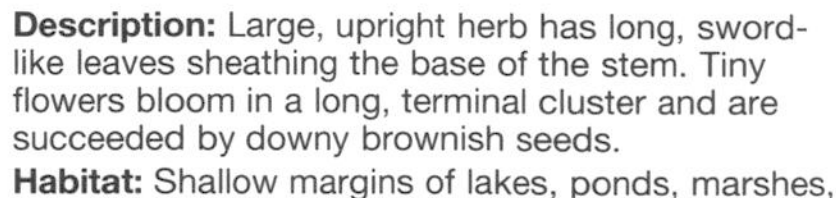

Cattail
Typha latifolia
To 10 ft. (3 m)

Description: Large, upright herb has long, sword-like leaves sheathing the base of the stem. Tiny flowers bloom in a long, terminal cluster and are succeeded by downy brownish seeds.
Habitat: Shallow margins of lakes, ponds, marshes, ditches.
Harvest: Shoots, roots, stalks, spikes.
Preparation: Young shoots can be eaten raw. Stalks can be peeled, boiled until tender. Green seed heads can be boiled and eaten like corn on the cob.
Comments: One of the most useful and widespread edible and medicinal plants.

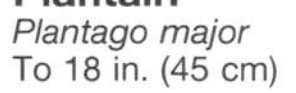
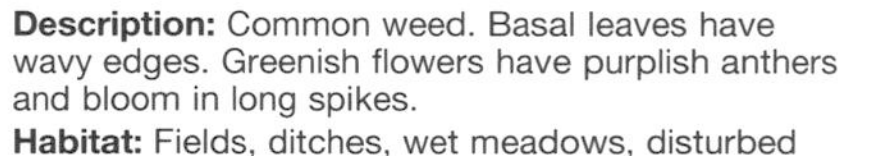

Plantain
Plantago major
To 18 in. (45 cm)

Description: Common weed. Basal leaves have wavy edges. Greenish flowers have purplish anthers and bloom in long spikes.
Habitat: Fields, ditches, wet meadows, disturbed areas.
Harvest: Leaves, seeds.
Preparation: Eat leaves raw or boiled or steep to make tea. Strip seeds from flower stalks, dry and grind into flour.
Comments: Rich in vitamins A, C and minerals.

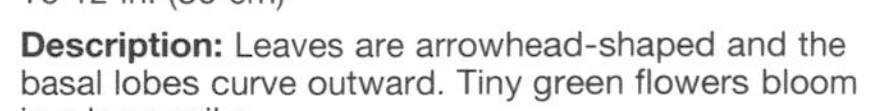

Sheep Sorrel
Rumex acetosella
To 12 in. (30 cm)

Description: Leaves are arrowhead-shaped and the basal lobes curve outward. Tiny green flowers bloom in a long spike.
Habitat: Disturbed areas, open sites with acidic soils.
Harvest: Leaves.
Preparation: Eat raw or boiled, or make a thirst-quenching, lemony tea.
Comments: Also called sour weed.

Nature's Supermarket

The cattail is one of the most widespread and useful wild edibles. The young shoots can be eaten raw or boiled. The root stock tubers can be boiled and eaten. The inner pith is edible raw or cooked. The pollen from seed heads can be collected and used as flour, and the young seed heads can be eaten like corn on the cob.

WILD EDIBLE PLANTS

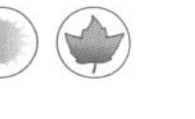

Dandelion
Taraxacum officinale
To 20 in. (50 cm)

Description: Long leaves are all basal and irregularly toothed. Puffy yellow flowerheads are succeeded by plume-tailed seeds that are spread by the wind.
Habitat: Fields, disturbed sites, roadsides, open areas.
Harvest: All parts of the plant are edible.
Preparation: Leaves can be used in salads or as a potherb. Dried flowers can be steeped to make tea. The root can be prepared like carrots or be dried and crushed to make a coffee substitute.
Comments: A rich source of vitamin A. The plant's coarsely toothed leaves give the plant its name which means 'lion's tooth.'

Nettle
Urtica spp.
To 7 ft. (2.1 m)

Description: Erect leafy plant is covered with stinging hairs that cause a burning sensation.
Habitat: Fields, meadows, woodlands, disturbed sites.
Harvest: Leaves, young shoots.
Preparation: To neutralize the stinging acid, simply boil in water.
Comments: Harvest with gloves on. An excellent source of vitamins A, B6, C, D, E, F, K as well as thiamin, riboflavin, niacin. One of the first plants to appear in spring. Dried nettle leaves are 40% protein.

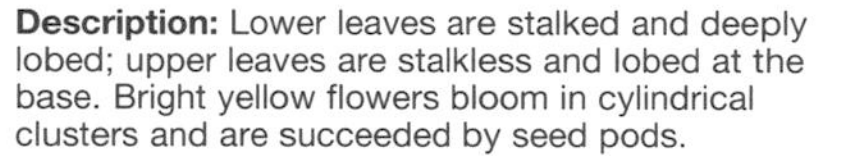

Wintercress
Barbarea vulgaris
To 28 in. (70 cm)

Description: Lower leaves are stalked and deeply lobed; upper leaves are stalkless and lobed at the base. Bright yellow flowers bloom in cylindrical clusters and are succeeded by seed pods.
Habitat: Fields, ditches, wet meadows.
Harvest: Leaves, buds, flowers.
Preparation: Leaves and flower buds can be eaten in salads and soups.
Comments: Leaves can be harvested throughout winter.

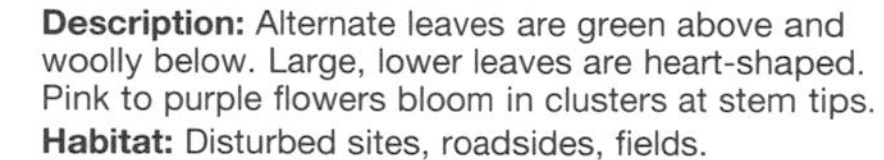

Burdock
Arctium spp.
To 6 ft. (1.8 m)

Description: Alternate leaves are green above and woolly below. Large, lower leaves are heart-shaped. Pink to purple flowers bloom in clusters at stem tips.
Habitat: Disturbed sites, roadsides, fields.
Harvest: Roots, leafstalks, young leaves.
Preparation: Peel roots and boil in two changes of water. Peel stalks and eat like celery. Eat leaves raw or boiled.
Comments: The prickly heads of this plant – burrs – attach readily to fur, feathers and clothing and aid in seed dispersal. The plant burrs were the inspiration for Velcro®.

The Importance of Charcoal

Charcoal is an indispensable resource in the case of accidental poisoning. Ground-up charcoal in water will induce vomiting when swallowed. The residual charcoal left in the stomach will absorb remaining toxins in the stomach.

WILD EDIBLE PLANTS

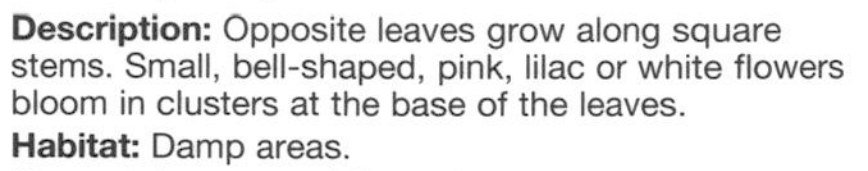

Wild Mint
Mentha arvensis
To 32 in. (80 cm)

Description: Opposite leaves grow along square stems. Small, bell-shaped, pink, lilac or white flowers bloom in clusters at the base of the leaves.
Habitat: Damp areas.
Harvest: Leaves and flower buds.
Preparation: Eat raw or boiled or use in tea.
Comments: The leaves have a strong minty, bitter flavor. Makes a good seasoning for meat.

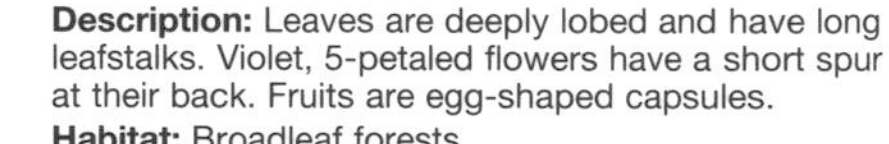
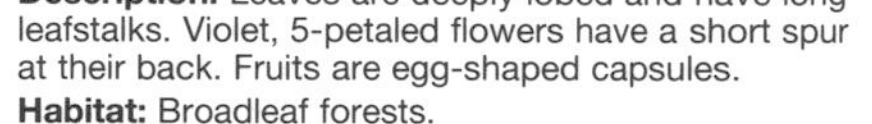

Violet
Viola spp.
To 16 in. (40 cm)

Description: Leaves are deeply lobed and have long leafstalks. Violet, 5-petaled flowers have a short spur at their back. Fruits are egg-shaped capsules.
Habitat: Broadleaf forests.
Harvest: Flowers, seed capsules, leaves.
Preparation: Eat raw or boiled. Grind seeds into flour.
Comments: Only harvest flowering plants so you identify them properly, the leaves mimic a number of poisonous species.

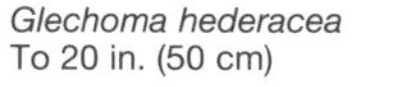

Gill-over-the-Ground
Glechoma hederacea
To 20 in. (50 cm)

Description: Creeping plant has kidney-shaped, opposite leaves with rounded, toothed edges. Blue to violet flowers are funnel-shaped and bloom in the spring.
Habitat: Disturbed sites, fields, shaded woods, roadsides.
Harvest: Leaves.
Preparation: Eat raw or boiled. Tea is rich in vitamin C.
Comments: Also called creeping Charlie and ground ivy.

Amaranth (Pigweed)
Amaranthus retroflexus
To 6.5 ft. (2 m)

Description: Coarse herb has long-stalked leaves that are widest near the base. Flowers bloom in in a dense, terminal cluster and are succeeded by capsule fruits.
Habitat: Waste areas, fields, roadsides.
Harvest: Leaves, seeds.
Preparation: Leaves should be boiled to remove oxalic acid (discard the water). Soft, fleshy top of the plant can be boiled and eaten like broccoli. Seeds are edible raw or toasted.
Comments: Often used to feed pigs and cattle.

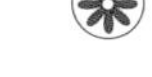
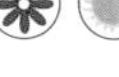

Field Lettuce
Valerianella locusta
To 5 in. (13 cm)

Description: Low-growing plant has deep green, rounded, spatulate leaves.
Habitat: Disturbed sites, fields, meadows, dry soils.
Harvest: Leaves.
Preparation: Eat raw or boiled.
Comments: Also called corn salad and lamb's lettuce, it is grown in warmer climates as a winter green. A good source of vitamins C, B6, B9, and E.

PREPARING WILD EDIBLES

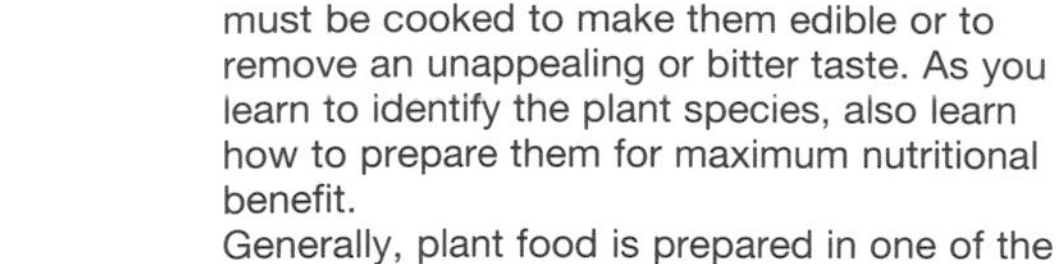
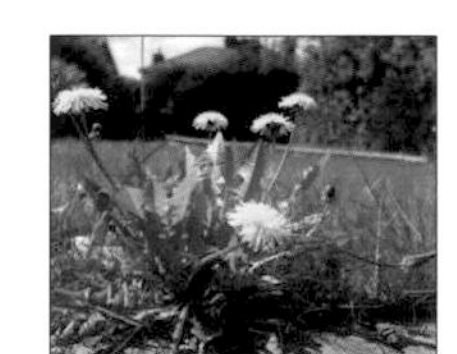
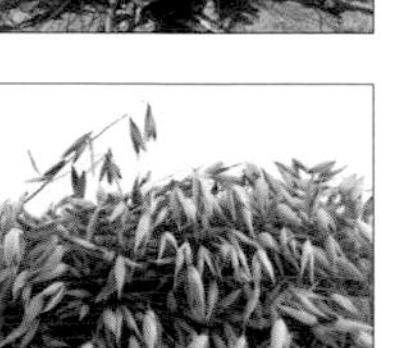
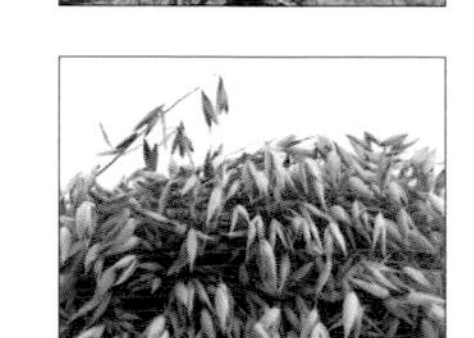
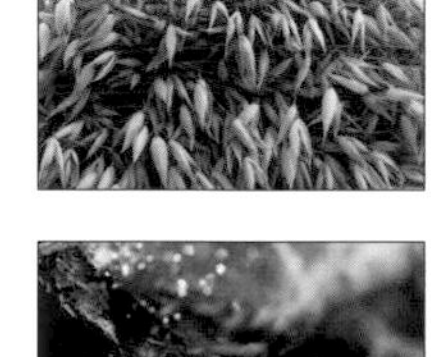
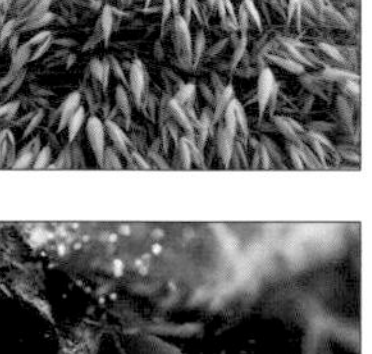
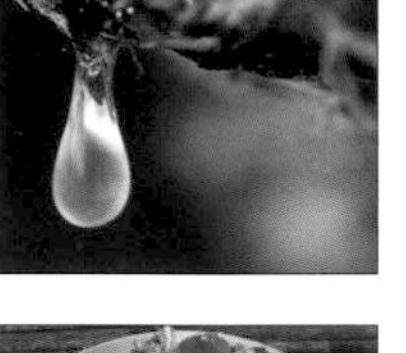
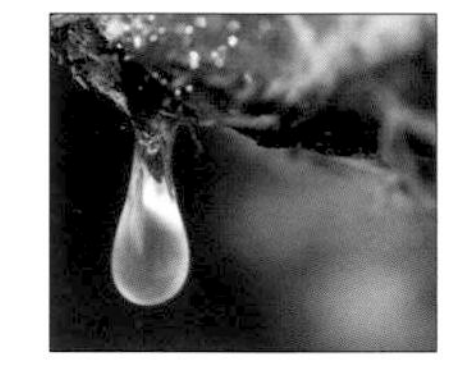

While some plants are edible raw, others must be cooked to make them edible or to remove an unappealing or bitter taste. As you learn to identify the plant species, also learn how to prepare them for maximum nutritional benefit.

Generally, plant food is prepared in one of the following ways: soaking, boiling, cooking, drying, or leaching.

- With leaves, stems and buds, boiling will remove bitterness. Certain plants need boiling in several changes of water to make them palatable. You should avoid boiling young leaves and shoots since this will destroy their texture and leach all the nutrients into the water (except plants that must be boiled to remove toxins). Coarser greens require longer cooking.
- Roots and tubers are generally boiled, baked or roasted and can be cooked like potatoes. Drying helps remove oxalates from some roots in the Arum (wild onion) family.
- Some nuts, such as acorns, need to be leached (strained through water) to remove the bitter taste. Others, such as chestnuts, are edible raw but taste better roasted.
- Grains and seeds can usually be eaten raw. Harvest grass grain by rubbing the seed heads between your hands or pound them with a rounded stick; toss the grains in the air to separate the wheat from the chaff. Dried grains should be ground up for better digestibility.
- Sap from trees such as maple, birch, walnuts and sycamores contain sugar – boiling the sap down makes condensed, energy-rich syrup.
- The flowers of many plants are edible including wild onions and garlic, dandelions, daisies, bee balm, chamomile, chicory, clover, hibiscus, lavender, lilac, mint, rose, sage, sunflower and violets.

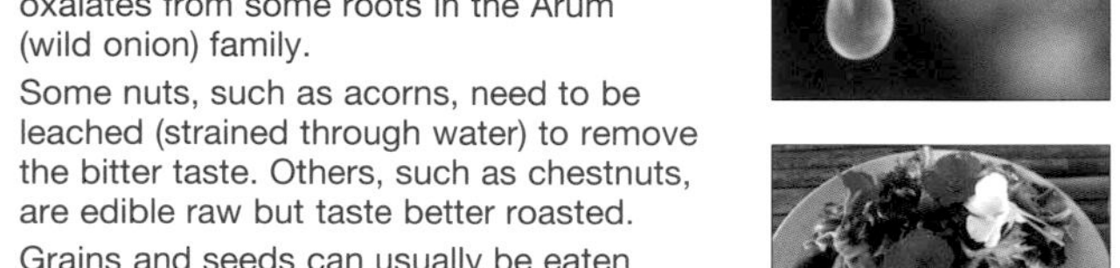
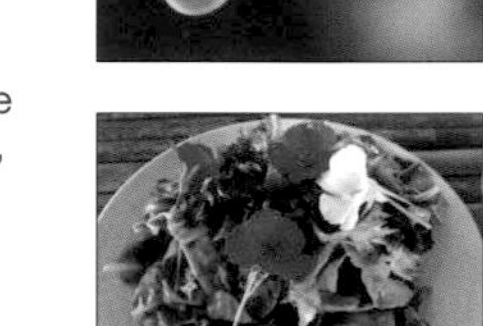
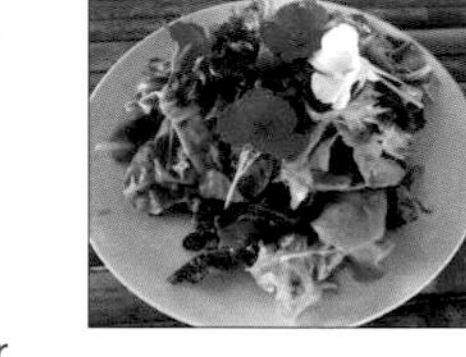
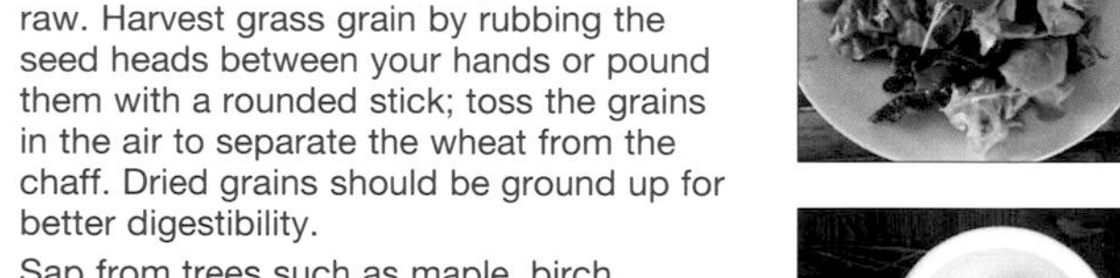
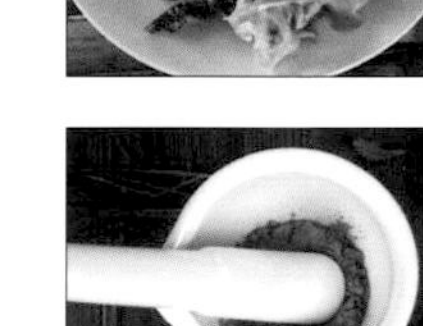
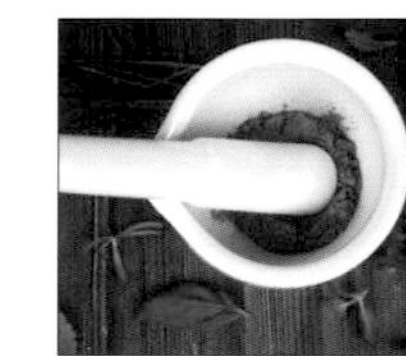
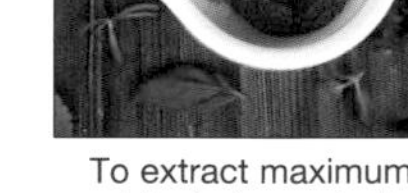

To extract maximum nutrients from plants, grind them into a pulp.

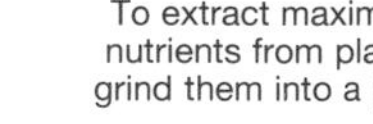
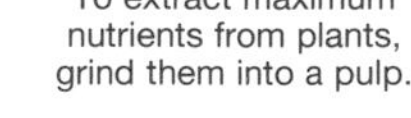

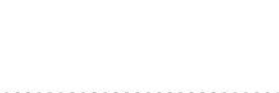

Making 'Teas'

Teas are made by steeping one handful of leaves (or needles), stems or fruits in one pint (2 cups) of hot water (preferably covered) for 10 minutes. Do not boil. Steeping the tea for longer periods of time will enhance the strength of the tea. When roots and bark are used in tea, they should be shredded or crushed thoroughly before steeping. Two very nutritious teas high in vitamin C can be made from pine needles and rose hips (the rounded fruits of rose bushes).

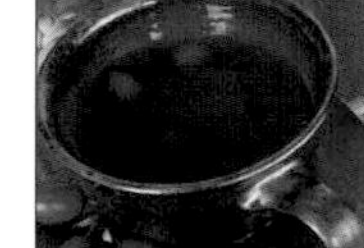
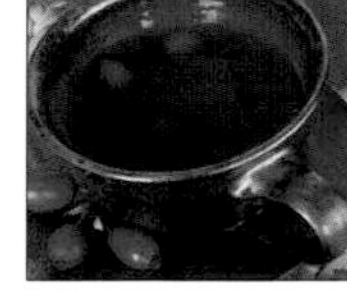
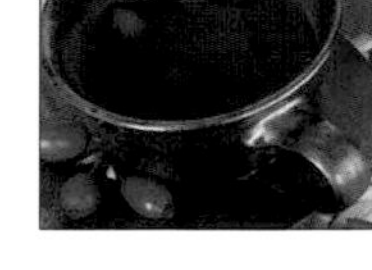
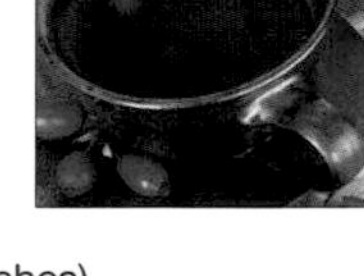